Obs and Gynae

PG Focus Series

Postpartum Hemorrhage and Internal Iliac Artery Ligation

Obs and Gynae

PG Focus Series

Postpartum Hemorrhage and Internal Iliac Artery Ligation

Editors

Niranjan Chavan

MD FICOG FCPS DGO DFP MICOG DICOG Diploma in Endoscopy (USA)
Professor and Unit Chief
Department of Obstetrics and Gynaecology
Lokmanya Tilak Medical College and General Hospital
Mumbai, Maharashtra, India

Komal N Chavan

MD DNB MNAMS FCPS DGO FICOG and Diploma in Reproductive Medicine (UK-SH Germany)
Senior Consultant and Unit Chief
Department of Obstetrics and Gynaecology
VN Desai Hospital
Mumbai, Maharashtra, India

Co-Editors

Darshana Ajmera

MBBS
Junior Resident 3
Department of Obstetrics and Gynaecology
Lokmanya Tilak Medical College and General Hospital
Mumbai, Maharashtra, India

Juili Tadkar

MBBS
Junior Resident 2
Department of Obstetrics and Gynaecology
Lokmanya Tilak Medical College and General Hospital
Mumbai, Maharashtra, India

JAYPEE

JAYPEE BROTHERS MEDICAL PUBLISHERS

The Health Sciences Publisher

New Delhi | London

Jaypee Brothers Medical Publishers (P) Ltd

Headquarters
Jaypee Brothers Medical Publishers (P) Ltd
EMCA House, 23/23-B
Ansari Road, Daryaganj
New Delhi 110 002, India
Landline: +91-11-23272143, +91-11-23272703
+91-11-23282021, +91-11-23245672
Email: jaypee@jaypeebrothers.com

Corporate Office
Jaypee Brothers Medical Publishers (P) Ltd
4838/24, Ansari Road, Daryaganj
New Delhi 110 002, India
Phone: +91-11-43574357
Fax: +91-11-43574314
Email: jaypee@jaypeebrothers.com

Overseas Office
JP Medical Ltd.
83, Victoria Street, London
SW1H 0HW (UK)
Phone: +44 20 3170 8910
Fax: +44 (0)20 3008 6180
Email: info@jpmedpub.com

Website: www.jaypeebrothers.com
Website: www.jaypeedigital.com

Inquiries for bulk sales may be solicited at: jaypee@jaypeebrothers.com

Obs and Gynae PG Focus Series: Postpartum Hemorrhage and Internal Iliac Artery Ligation

First Edition: **2025**

ISBN: 978-93-6616-510-3

Printed in India

Preface

Postpartum hemorrhage (PPH) remains a leading cause of maternal morbidity and mortality worldwide, despite significant advances in obstetric care. Managing severe PPH effectively requires prompt decision-making and expertise in life-saving techniques. Internal iliac artery ligation (IIAL) is a critical surgical intervention that has proven to be highly effective in controlling intractable hemorrhage while preserving future fertility.

This manual is designed to serve as a comprehensive guide for practitioners seeking to master the management of PPH, with a particular emphasis on the application of internal iliac artery ligation. Central to this approach is the innovative use of *Chavan's Internal Iliac Artery Ligation Forceps (CIIALF),* a groundbreaking instrument that simplifies the technical challenges of IIAL, enhances precision, and reduces procedure time. The CIIALF has revolutionized the management of PPH, making this life-saving procedure more accessible and efficient for practitioners worldwide.

The manual addresses fundamental topics such as the pathophysiology and risk factors of PPH, a detailed step-by-step approach to internal iliac artery ligation, and comprehensive guidance on the design, functionality, and application of the CIIALF. Practical insights are provided to address challenges encountered during the procedure, minimize complications, and optimize outcomes, particularly in high-risk or resource-limited settings.

By emphasizing the importance of *Chavan's Internal Iliac Artery Ligation Forceps,* this resource not only highlights a pivotal advancement in surgical instrumentation but also underscores its potential to significantly reduce maternal mortality and morbidity associated with PPH.

We hope this manual serves as an invaluable resource, empowering obstetricians to confidently manage PPH and utilize cutting-edge tools like the CIIALF to deliver safer, more effective care. Through knowledge, skill, and innovation, we aim to advance maternal health and save lives.

Editors
Niranjan Chavan
Komal N Chavan

Co-Editors
Darshana Ajmera
Juili Tadkar

Acknowledgments

With immense gratitude, we express our sincere thanks to all those who contributed to the completion of *Postpartum Hemorrhage and Internal Iliac Artery Ligation*. This endeavor would not have been possible without the encouragement and support of many individuals.

We extend our deepest thanks to all the authors and co-authors for sharing their expertise and their commitment to producing a resource of the highest standards.

Our heartfelt appreciation goes to our mentors and colleagues, whose valuable insights and guidance inspired the structure and content of this book. Their expertise and shared experiences have significantly enriched its scope.

To our families and friends: Your unwavering support, patience, and encouragement during the demanding phases of this project have been our greatest strength.

We would also like to acknowledge Dr Niranjan Chavan unit members—Dr Deepali (Associate Professor), Dr Swara (Assistant Professor), Dr Vishwaja (Assistant Professor), and all the junior residents—Dr Shruti Rane, Dr Radhika Bhutada, Dr Monika Dhauchak, and Dr Rutuja Mohite for their dedication, time, and hard work. Their efforts, in addition to managing their hectic schedules, were instrumental in bringing this book to life.

We especially appreciate the constant support and encouragement of Shri Jitendar P Vij (Group Chairman) and Mr Ankit Vij (Managing Director) of M/s Jaypee Brothers Medical Publishers (P) Ltd, New Delhi, India, in publishing the book and their associates, particularly Ms Chetna Malhotra (Senior Director—Professional Publishing, Marketing, and Business Development), Ms Kritika Dua (Senior Commissiong Editor), Mr Pragati Singh and Mr Priyansh Saxena (Development Editors), who have been prompt, efficient, and most helpful.

Lastly, to the readers and practitioners of obstetrics and gynaecology, we hope this book serves as a valuable resource, contributing to the betterment of patient care and surgical practice.

Thank you all for being a part of this journey.

Contents

CHAPTER 1

Introduction

Postpartum hemorrhage (PPH) remains a leading cause of maternal mortality and morbidity globally, accounting for approximately a quarter of maternal deaths worldwide. Its incidence in developed countries has been increasing, highlighting the ongoing challenge in managing this severe complication.

BRIEF HISTORICAL OVERVIEW

Postpartum hemorrhage (PPH), the excessive bleeding following childbirth, has been a significant concern throughout human history. The management of PPH has evolved significantly over time, reflecting advances in medical knowledge, technology, and clinical practice.

Historically, PPH was a leading cause of maternal mortality, particularly in the absence of effective interventions. Ancient medical texts from various cultures, such as Egyptian, Greek, and Indian, document attempts to manage PPH using a range of methods, including herbal remedies, uterine massage, and compression techniques. However, these methods often proved ineffective in controlling severe bleeding.

During the middle ages & renaissance, obstetrical practices continued to develop, but effective management of PPH remained elusive. It was not until the 19th century that significant progress was made in understanding the causes of PPH and developing more effective interventions. The introduction of obstetrical forceps, improved techniques for delivering the placenta, and advances in surgical skills helped reduce the incidence of PPH and improve outcomes for women.[1]

In the late 19th and early 20th centuries, the discovery of uterotonics, drugs that stimulate uterine contractions, revolutionized the management of PPH. Ergot alkaloids, such as ergonovine, were among the first uterotonics used to control postpartum bleeding. Later, synthetic oxytocin became the primary pharmacological agent for preventing and treating PPH, as it was found to be highly effective in inducing uterine contractions and reducing blood loss.

In the early 1950s, American biochemist Vincent du Vigneaud **(Fig. 1)** discovered that oxytocin is composed of nine amino acids and determined its sequence. In 1953, he successfully synthesized oxytocin, making it the first polypeptide hormone to be artificially created—a breakthrough that earned him the Nobel Prize in Chemistry in 1955. Synthetic oxytocin soon became

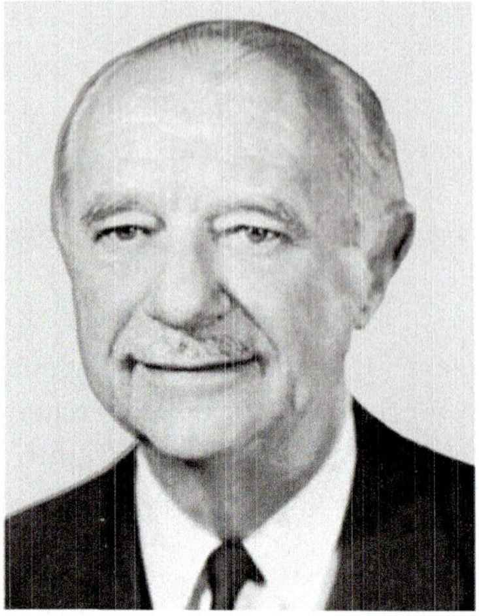

Fig. 1: Dr Vincent du Vigneaud.
Source: Britannica. Vincent du Vigneaud. [online] Available from https://www.britannica.com/biography/Vincent-du-Vigneaud. [Last accessed November, 2024]

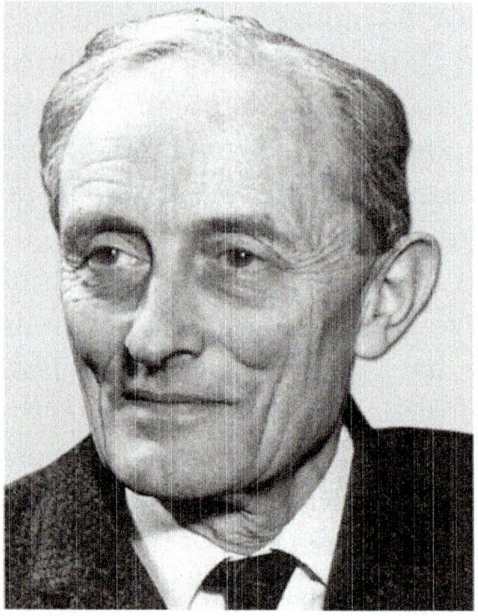

Fig. 2: Dr John Chassar Moir.
Source: National Library of Medicine. Dr John Chassar Moir. [online] Available from https://cdn.ncbi.nlm.nih.gov/pmc/blobs/a067/1721462/2b3c3447ebc3/02017.f1.jpg. [Last accessed November, 2024]

widely used in obstetrics for labor induction or maintenance, postpartum bleeding control, and to promote milk letdown for breastfeeding.

In the early 1930s, Dr John Chassar Moir **(Fig. 2)** led research that led to the discovery and identification of ergometrine, the active water-soluble component of rye ergot. Its application in preventing and controlling postpartum hemorrhage has saved countless lives over the years. He stated that, the primary use of ergometrine is in the prevention and treatment of postpartum hemorrhage, where its effects are most beneficial. If the uterus remains overly relaxed after the placenta is delivered, administering ergometrine—1 mg orally or 0.5 mg by injection—will promptly induce a strong contraction of the organ.[2]

The development of modern obstetric techniques, such as active management of the third stage of labor (AMTSL), also played a crucial role in reducing the incidence of PPH. The ability to quickly provide blood products, such as packed red blood cells and fresh frozen plasma, has saved countless lives by restoring circulating blood volume and preventing hemorrhagic shock.[3]

REFERENCES

1. Begley CM, Gyte GM, Devane D, McGuire W, Weeks A, Biesty LM. Active versus expectant management for women in the third stage of labour. Cochrane Database Syst Rev. 2019;2(2):CD007412.
2. Dunn PM. John Chassar Moir (1900-1977) and the discovery of ergometrine. Arch Dis Child Fetal Neonatal Ed. 2002;87(2):F152-4.
3. Meh C, Sharma A, Ram U, Fadel S, Correa N, Snelgrove J, et al. Trends in maternal mortality in India over two decades in nationally representative surveys. BJOG Int J Obstet Gynaecol. 2022;129(4):550-61.

2 CHAPTER Etiology

INTRODUCTION

The most common cause of postpartum hemorrhage (PPH) is uterine atony, which occurs when the myometrium fails to contract and retract after delivery, preventing the cessation of bleeding at the placental site.

Atonic PPH accounts for 80% of all primary PPH cases. Other causes include genital tract trauma, retained placental tissue, and, less frequently, coagulopathy **(Table 1 and Fig. 1)**.

RISK FACTORS

- Placenta previa
- Abruptio placenta
- Multiple pregnancy
- Preeclampsia/hypertension
- Asian ethnicity
- Previous PPH
- Obesity (body mass index >35)
- Anemia (Hb <9.0 g)
- Induced labor
- Emergency/elective caesarean section
- Mediolateral episiotomy
- Operative vaginal delivery
- Big baby weight >4 kg

TABLE 1: The 4 Ts' causes of PPH.

Four "Ts" cause	*Approximate incidence (%)*
Tone—atonic uterus	70
Trauma—lacerations, hematomas, inversion, rupture	10
Tissue—retained tissue	20
Thrombin—coagulopathies	<1

(PPH: postpartum hemorrhage)
Source: José F, De E, Franklin EDLH, Muñoz DME, Alexander J, Mogollón E, et al. Effectiveness of Hayman's Compressive Suture in the Management of Postpartum Hemorrhage. 2019;3(4):285-90.

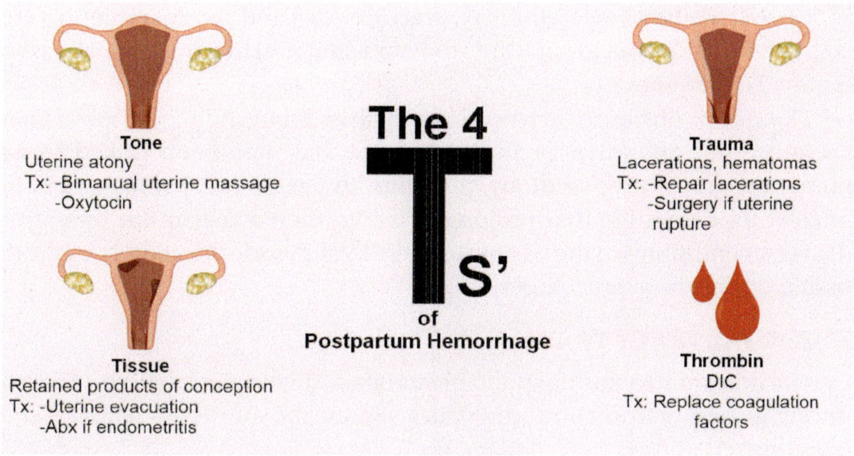

Fig. 1: Causes of PPH. (PPH: postpartum hemorrhage)
Source: Tintinalli JE, Ma OJ, Yealy DM, Meckler GD, Stapczynski JS, Cline DM, et al. Tintinalli's Emergency Medicine: A Comprehensive Study Guide, 9th edition. New York: McGraw Hill; 2020.

- Prolonged labor >12 hours
- Age >40 years
- Pyrexia in labor

UTERINE ATONY

Uterine atony is the most common cause of PPH, accounting for 70–80% of cases. During pregnancy, maternal blood volume increases by approximately 50% (from 4 L to 6 L), while uterine blood flow at term reaches 500–800 mL per minute, which represents 10–15% of cardiac output. The uterine artery branches that supply blood to the placental bed pass through myometrial fibers arranged in longitudinal, transverse, and oblique patterns. After childbirth, the contraction and retraction of these "criss-cross" fibers cause placental separation and the constriction of blood vessels, leading to the occlusion of blood flow. This natural arrangement, often referred to as "living ligatures" or "physiologic sutures," allows the uterus to "clamp down" on the blood vessels supplying the placental bed, reducing blood loss.[1]

Uterine atony occurs when this living ligature system fails to contract and retract properly after delivery, leaving the placental bed supplied by "unclamped" uterine blood vessels, resulting in continued bleeding.

Unlike certain conditions like placental abnormalities that can be detected during pregnancy, uterine atony is difficult to predict. Various risk factors have been identified in previous studies, including uterine overdistension (e.g., multiple pregnancies, polyhydramnios), rapid or prolonged labor, oxytocin stimulation, and obesity. Recent research has shown that maternal race/ethnicity, preeclampsia, and chorioamnionitis are consistent risk factors for uterine atony in women delivering vaginally who required treatment.

The rise in obstetric interventions, such as labor induction, caesarean sections, and operative vaginal deliveries, has also been linked to an increased risk of uterine atony, although the exact mechanisms remain unclear. It is possible that prolonged labor, often a reason for operative delivery, contributes to the risk of atonic PPH, alongside the added trauma to tissues during these procedures.[2]

GENITAL TRACT TRAUMA

Genital tract trauma during spontaneous or assisted vaginal delivery, or even during a caesarean section, can cause significant soft tissue damage and blood vessel rupture.

Trauma accounts for 10–15% of PPH cases and includes conditions such as genital tract lacerations, uterine rupture, and uterine inversion. It is estimated that over 85% of women who have a vaginal birth experience some degree of perineal trauma, and 60%–70% of these women require suturing.

In some cases, bleeding caused by genital tract trauma may not be immediately visible, as it can result in paravaginal or broad ligament hematomas. These hematomas should be suspected when severe pain is present or when changes in vital signs are out of proportion to the visible blood loss. Hematomas can be localized to the vulva or extend to the infralevator and supralevator regions.[3]

RETAINED PLACENTAL TISSUE

Retained tissue refers to blood clots, retained placenta, cotyledons, and membranes. The mean duration of time from delivery of the fetus until placental expulsion is usually 8–9 minutes. If this duration increases, then the risk of PPH may also increase as the uterus is unable to contract and retract effectively in the presence of the placenta and membranes.

The risk of PPH is estimated to double after 10 minutes. Retained placenta refers to a failure of the placenta to be expelled within 30 minutes after birth and this occurs in <3% of all vaginal deliveries. One management option for retained placenta is to inject the umbilical vein with 20 mL of a solution of 0.9% saline and 20 units of oxytocin.

However, recent evidence has shown that this approach does not reduce the need for manual removal of the placenta (MROP) compared with injecting saline alone. MROP should be performed under suitable analgesia in the operation theater to arrest ongoing bleeding.

COAGULOPATHY

Coagulopathy refers to disorders of the blood's coagulation system, which can, though rarely, lead to primary PPH. Coagulation abnormalities should be considered in cases where the usual treatments for PPH are ineffective, especially if the uterus is well contracted.

Common causes of PPH due to coagulopathy include idiopathic thrombocytopenic purpura (ITP), thrombotic thrombocytopenic purpura (TTP), von Willebrand disease (vWF), and hemophilia. Acquired coagulation disorders may develop in association with conditions like severe preeclampsia, HELLP syndrome (hemolysis, elevated liver enzymes, and low platelet count), or as a result of disseminated intravascular coagulation (DIC). DIC can occur in the context of severe preeclampsia, amniotic fluid embolism, sepsis, placental abruption, or a retained dead fetus.[4]

CAUSES OF SECONDARY POSTPARTUM HEMORRHAGE

- Products of conception—retained placental tissue and membrane
- Endometritis
- Placental site trophoblastic tumor (gestational trophoblastic tissue)
- Arteriovenous malformations (e.g., pseudoaneurysm of the uterine artery)

REFERENCES

1. Lalonde A, FIGO Safe Motherhood and Newborn Health (SMNH) Committee. Prevention and treatment of postpartum hemorrhage in low-resource settings. Int J Gynecol Obstet. 2012;117(2):108-18.
2. Weiskopf RB, Feiner J, Hopf H, Viele MK, Watson JJ, Lieberman J, et al. Heart rate increases linearly in response to acute isovolemic anemia. Transfusion (Paris). 2003;43(2):235-40.
3. Nygaard KK, Wilder M, Berkson J. The relation between viscosity of the blood and the relative volume of erythrocytes (hematocrit value). Am J Physiol-Leg Content. 1935;114(1):128-31.
4. Whittaker SR, Winton FR. The apparent viscosity of blood flowing in the isolated hindlimb of the dog, and its variation with corpuscular concentration. J Physiol. 1933;78(4):339-69.

3

CHAPTER

Diagnosis of Postpartum Hemorrhage

INTRODUCTION

Postpartum hemorrhage (PPH) is a leading cause of maternal mortality, necessitating accurate assessment and timely intervention. Traditional methods like visual blood loss estimation often underestimate the severity of hemorrhage, particularly at higher volumes.

Direct measurement, using graduated containers or weighing surgical swabs and pads, offers greater accuracy but can be influenced by contamination from fluids like urine and amniotic fluid. Clinical tools such as the Shock Index (SI), which assesses heart rate relative to blood pressure, and early warning score systems, which evaluate multiple vital signs, provide critical insights for identifying and managing severe PPH.

Timely recognition and response, particularly during the "golden first hour," are essential to prevent life-threatening complications. This chapter focuses on evidence-based tools and techniques that enhance the assessment and management of PPH, improving maternal outcomes.

VISUAL ESTIMATION OF BLOOD LOSS

Most clinicians attempt to visually estimate the amount of blood loss during postpartum hemorrhage (PPH), but this method is known to be highly inaccurate, with significant variation between and within observers. Its accuracy diminishes as the volume of blood loss increases. A study by Prasertcharoensuk and colleagues found that visual estimates of blood loss during vaginal births underestimated the incidence of PPH by 89%. Obstetricians typically estimate blood loss by observing the amount collected in obstetric drapes, but blood is often mixed with urine and absorbed by surgical sponges/swabs. Visual assessment has been shown to underestimate postpartum blood loss by 33–50% when compared to objective methods like photospectrometry **(Fig. 1)**.

DIRECT MEASUREMENT

Direct measurement is one of the oldest and most accurate methods of determining blood loss. This method requires multiple containers to collect the blood and a graduated container to measure the volume. It can be used regardless of the woman's position or location during birth. However, contamination with amniotic fluid and urine can complicate measurement. Surgical swabs, pads, and drapes can also be weighed before and after use to

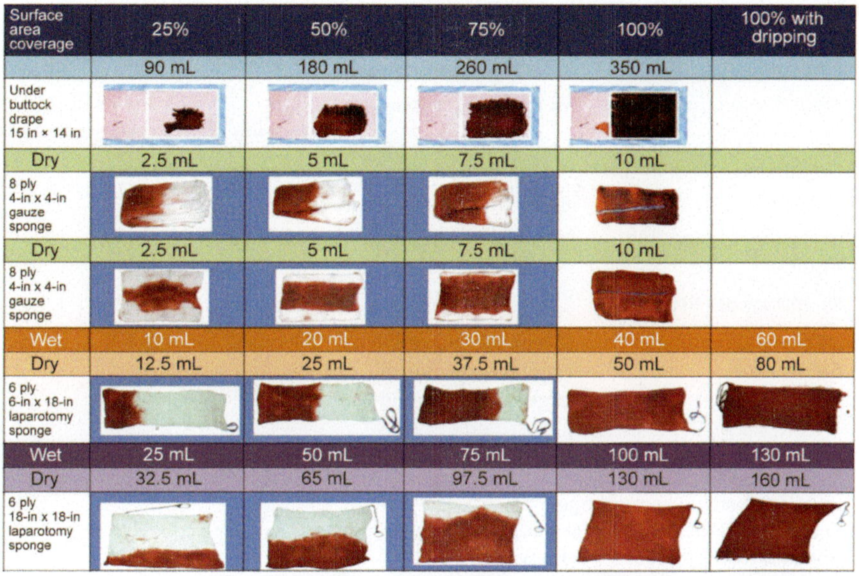

Fig. 1: Visual assessment to underestimate postpartum blood loss.
Source: Phutchjirah C, Poolnoi P. Using blood loss pictogram for visual blood loss estimation in cesarean section. J Med Assoc Thai. 2012;95(4):550-6.

calculate blood loss based on the difference in weight, a method commonly used in operating theaters. This approach should be performed shortly after birth to prevent drying and evaporation, which can affect accuracy.[1]

CLINICAL TOOLS FOR EARLY DETECTION OF SEVERE POSTPARTUM HEMORRHAGE

Shock Index

The shock index (SI) is used in intensive care units and trauma centers to estimate blood loss. It is calculated by dividing heart rate (HR) by systolic blood pressure (SBP), with a normal range between 0.5 and 0.7. In cases of significant hemorrhage, the heart rate increases and the SBP decreases, causing the SI to rise. An SI above 0.9–1.1 may indicate the need for intensive resuscitation. Recently, there has been interest in determining normal and abnormal values for an "obstetric shock index" (OSI). A preliminary study suggests that a normal OSI during pregnancy is 0.7–0.8, and an OSI greater than 1 signals massive obstetric hemorrhage, which requires blood transfusions in 80% of cases.

EARLY WARNING SCORE SYSTEM

Severe PPH can lead to cardiovascular compromise, requiring rapid resuscitative efforts. This should be initiated before blood loss exceeds one-third of the woman's total blood volume (calculated as weight in kg × 90 mL

TABLE 1: Risk assessment tool.

Low risk	*Medium risk*	*High risk*
Singleton pregnancy	Multiple gestation	Placenta previa, increta, percreta
No previous uterine surgery	Previous uterine surgeries	Bleeding at admission
No history of bleeding disorder	Magnesium sulfate use	Known coagulopathy
No history of PPH	Chorioamnionitis	HCT (hematocrit) <30
≤4 previous vaginal deliveries	More than four previous vaginal deliveries of large uterine fibroids	Platelet <100,000
	Prolonged use of oxytocin	

(PPH: postpartum hemorrhage)
Source: PQCNC. Updates. [online] Available from https://www.pqcnc.org/initiatives/updates/13805. [Last accessed November, 2024]

during pregnancy), or when blood loss is greater than 1,000 mL or there is a noticeable change in hemodynamic status. Early warning score systems were developed to help recognize life-threatening conditions earlier. These scores are based on factors such as SBP, temperature, pulse, respiratory rate, and mental status.

In a study involving 702 low-risk obstetric patients admitted to intensive care units, the early warning score system had an area under the curve of 0.84 (0.75–0.92) for predicting maternal death. Similar studies have shown comparable results, distinguishing women with adverse outcomes from those without.

The concept of the "golden first hour" emphasizes the importance of initiating resuscitation within this time to maximize survival before metabolic acidosis occurs. This has led to the development of the "rule of 30," which helps assess the severity of hemorrhage and shock. When a woman loses 30% of her blood volume, her SBP may drop by 30 mm Hg, her HR may increase by 30 bpm, her respiratory rate may exceed 30 breaths per minute, and her hemoglobin or hematocrit may decrease by 30%. Additionally, urinary output is likely to fall below 30 mL/hour due to peripheral shutdown. One or more of these signs can indicate moderate shock and the need for urgent intervention[2] **(Table 1)**.

SIGNS AND SYMPTOMS

The severity of symptoms and signs observed during PPH is directly related to the extent of ongoing blood loss. Different levels of shock have been described

TABLE 2: Obstetric shock index.

Shock index to mortality rates			
	Shock index	***Mortality rate***	***Blood products***
No shock	<0.6	10.9% mortality	1 unit
Mild shock	≥0.6 to <1.0	↓	2.8 unit
Moderate shock	≥1.0 to <1.4		9.9 unit
Severe shock	≥1.4	39.8% mortality	21.4 unit

Source: Shertz M. Shock Index: a more sophisticated determinant of hypovolemic shock. [online] Available from https://www.crisis-medicine.com/shock-index/. [Last accessed November, 2024]

based on the volume of blood lost. The obstetric shock index (OSI) **(Table 2)** can help identify even subtle increases in heart rate, which may signal the early stages of shock. Additionally, intense peripheral vasoconstriction diverts blood from nonessential organs to vital ones, potentially causing an increase in diastolic blood pressure (DBP) and resulting in a narrower "pulse pressure."

REFERENCES

1. Wohner N, Sótonyi P, Machovich R, Szabó L, Tenekedjiev K, Silva MMCG, et al. Lytic resistance of fibrin containing red blood cells. Arterioscler Thromb Vasc Biol. 2011;31(10):2306-13.
2. Anand A, Feffer SE. Hematocrit and bleeding time: an update. South Med J. 1994;87(3):299-301.

CHAPTER 4

Management of Postpartum Hemorrhage: Medical

INTRODUCTION

Managing postpartum hemorrhage (PPH) requires a logical and systematic approach to save lives **(Flowchart 1)**. Confidential inquiries into maternal deaths have consistently highlighted the issue of "too little, too late" as a significant factor contributing to deaths from PPH. Therefore, management should focus on rapid identification and treatment of the specific underlying cause, effective communication, thorough assessment, and the involvement of a multidisciplinary team for resuscitation, monitoring, and management of women who experience massive blood loss.

Chandraharan and Arulkumaran introduced the "HEMOSTASIS" algorithm **(Fig. 1)** to guide the systematic management of PPH. A recent study indicated that using the HEMOSTASIS algorithm provided a timely and structured approach to managing PPH, successfully controlling over 90% of cases involving massive blood loss. In this study, the risk of peripartum hysterectomy in cases of severe PPH was reduced to less than 2%.[1]

Effective communication is essential in managing PPH and requires the involvement of a multidisciplinary team, including senior obstetricians, midwives, anesthetists, and haematologist. It is also important to keep the woman and her family informed, as much as possible, so they can make informed decisions, especially if life-saving interventions like peripartum hysterectomy are being considered.

Assessment should include an evaluation of the woman's overall condition, estimated blood loss (EBL), the identification of the cause of PPH, and monitoring of vital signs.

Resuscitation focuses on ensuring the ABCs:

- *Airway and breathing*: Ensure an open airway and administer oxygen at 8–12 L/min via a face mask, regardless of the woman's oxygen saturation level. If the airway is compromised, anesthesia support should be called immediately.
- *Circulation*: Establish two large-bore (14-gauge) IV lines for rapid fluid administration and simultaneously draw 20 mL of blood for diagnostic tests, including full blood count, urea and electrolytes, coagulation profile, and cross-matching for four units of blood. Blood pressure, pulse, and respiratory rate should be monitored every 15 minutes.

Flowchart 1: Medical management of PPH.

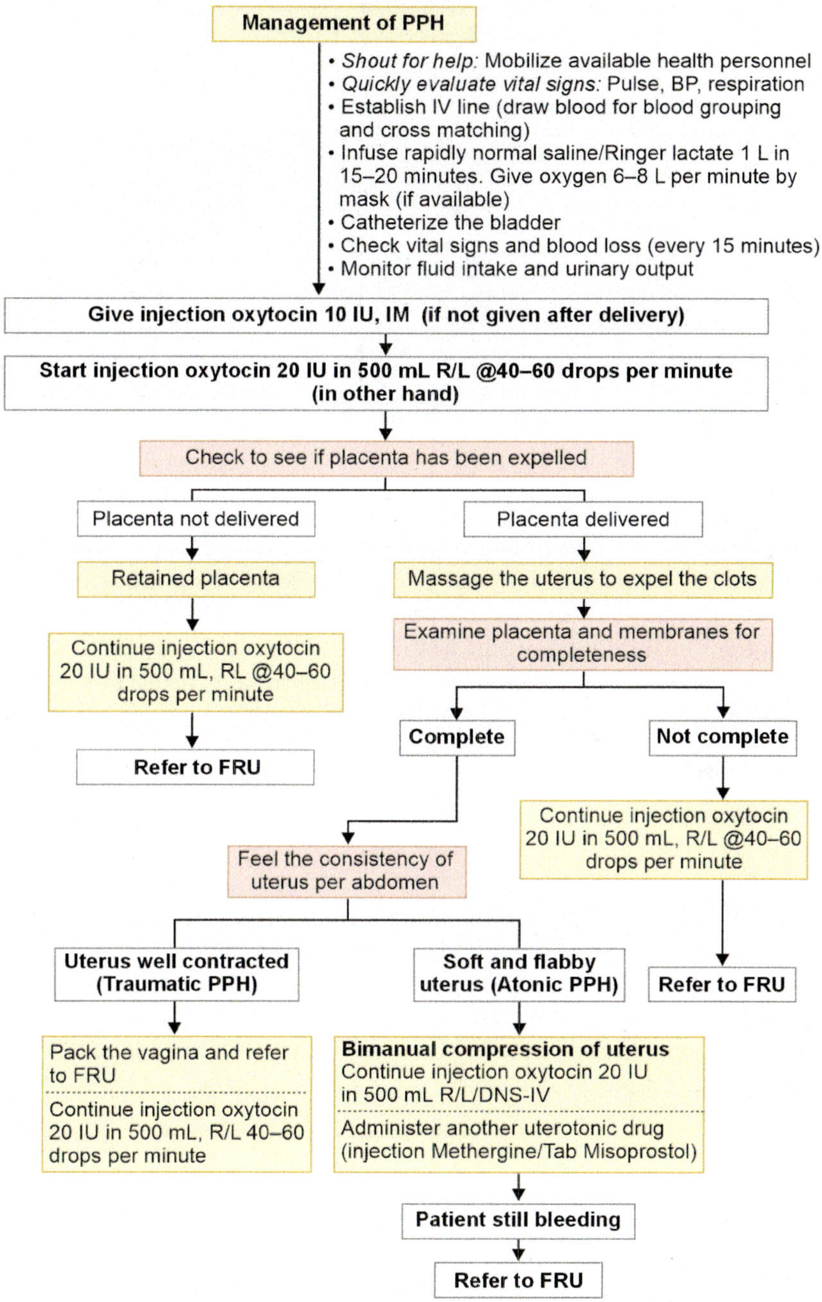

(FRU: first referral unit; PPH: postpartum hemorrhage)

Source: https://x.com/USAID_RMNCHA/status/820519217657159681

- H—Ask for help
- A—Assess (vitals, blood loss) and resuscitate
- E—Establish etiology (tone, tissue, trauma, thrombin)
  - —Ecbolics (syntometrine, ergometrine)
  - —Ensure availability of blood
- M—Massage the uterus
- O—Oxytocin infusion and prostaglandin
- S—Shift to operating theater
  - —Bimanual compression nonpneumatic or pneumatic antishock garment
- T—Tissue and trauma to be excluded
- A—Apply compression sutures
- S—Systematic pelvic devascularization
- I—Interventional radiology
- S—Subtotal/total hysterectomy

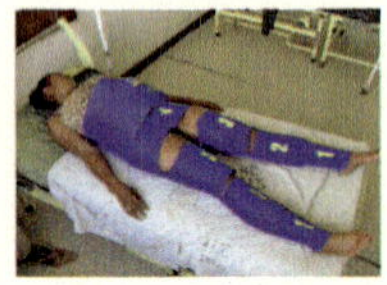

Fig. 1: "HEMOSTASIS" algorithm.
Source: Chandraharan E, Krishna A. Diagnosis and management of postpartum haemorrhage. BMJ. 2017;358:j3875.

It is recommended to have a dedicated PPH trolley stocked with the necessary drugs and equipment for initial management. If massive blood loss (over 2 L) is suspected, a "Massive Obstetric Hemorrhage Protocol," such as declaring a "Code Blue," should be activated immediately. Additional interventions include lowering the head of the bed to enhance venous return and cerebral circulation and preventing hypothermia by using warmed air blankets and prewarmed fluids during resuscitation.[2]

FLUID THERAPY

The primary goal of fluid therapy is to restore blood volume, maintain oxygen-carrying capacity, and replenish depleted coagulation factors. While the ideal replacement is blood and blood products, until these become available, a rapid infusion of prewarmed crystalloids (such as 2 L of Hartmann's solution) and colloids (1.5 L) should be administered.

If, after 3.5 L of fluid resuscitation, fully cross-matched blood is still unavailable and the bleeding continues or the patient's condition worsens, uncross-matched group-specific blood or O RhD-negative blood may be administered as clinically necessary.

Platelet concentrates should be given if platelet count is <50,000.

When 4 units of red cells have been transfused or if activated partial thromboplastin time (aPTT) or prothrombin time (PT) >1.5 then 4 units of fresh frozen plasma (FFP) should be administered.[3]

MECHANICAL METHODS

If the placenta has been delivered and there is persistent bleeding from a boggy (i.e., atonic) uterus, uterine fundal massage or bimanual uterine compression should be performed to stimulate uterine contractions.

This "uterine massage" aids in both the contraction and retraction of the uterus and helps expel blood clots.

In some cases, the uterine fundus may be firm and contracted while the lower segment remains dilated and atonic. In such situations, the approach involves manually removing any clots and applying bimanual compression to reduce blood flow while waiting for uterotonic agents to take effect. Additionally, inserting an indwelling urinary catheter to empty the bladder can help promote uterine contraction and retraction.

PHARMACOLOGICAL METHODS

Uterotonic Agents

Oxytocin (Syntocinon) 5 IU via slow IV injection is the first-line treatment for atonic PPH. It can be combined with 0.5 mg of ergometrine (Syntometrine). Oxytocin works by stimulating rhythmic contractions in the fundal myometrium, which constricts the spiral arteries and reduces uterine blood flow. Alternatively, a slow IV/IM injection of 0.5 mg of ergometrine can be administered, which induces a generalized tetanic contraction of the myometrium, affecting both the upper and lower uterine segments. However, ergometrine can cause intense peripheral vasoconstriction and increase blood pressure, making it contraindicated in women with hypertension or cardiac conditions.

If the bleeding persists, an oxytocin infusion should be started at a rate of 125 mL/h (10 units of oxytocin/h) by adding 40 IU of Syntocinon to 500 mL of Hartmann solution.

Prostaglandins

Prostaglandins are used to enhance uterine contractions and promote vasoconstriction. The most commonly used is carboprost (Hemabate), a 15-methyl prostaglandin F2α. Carboprost 0.25 mg (250 mcg) can be given intramuscularly and repeated every 15 minutes for up to eight doses (maximum 2 mg). Although effective in 87% of patients, carboprost is contraindicated in individuals with bronchial asthma due to the risk of bronchoconstriction. Caution is also needed for intramyometrial injections, as accidental injection into the uterine veins can lead to maternal cardiac arrest.

Misoprostol is another effective prostaglandin for treating atonic PPH, though it often causes side effects like nausea, vomiting, and diarrhea, which may limit its use in some settings. It can be administered sublingually, orally, vaginally, or rectally, with doses ranging from 200 to 1000 mcg. The International Federation of Gynaecology and Obstetrics (FIGO) recommends a sublingual dose of 800 mcg (four 200 mcg tablets). Carbetocin, a long-acting oxytocin derivative, is not currently supported by evidence as a first-line treatment for PPH.[4]

REFERENCES

1. Aarts PA, van den Broek SA, Prins GW, Kuiken GD, Sixma JJ, Heethaar RM. Blood platelets are concentrated near the wall and red blood cells, in the center in flowing blood. Arterioscler Dallas Tex. 1988;8(6):819-24.
2. Nair M, Choudhury MK, Choudhury SS, Kakoty SD, Sarma UC, Webster P, et al. Association between maternal anaemia and pregnancy outcomes: a cohort study in Assam, India. BMJ Glob Health. 2016;1(1):e000026.
3. Lavallée JF, Gray TA, Dumville J, Russell W, Cullum N. The effects of care bundles on patient outcomes: a systematic review and meta-analysis. Implement Sci IS. 2017;12(1):142.
4. Gallos I, Devall A, Martin J, Middleton L, Beeson L, Galadanci H, et al. Randomized Trial of Early Detection and Treatment of Postpartum Hemorrhage. N Engl J Med. 2023;389(1):11-21.

5

CHAPTER

Management of Postpartum Hemorrhage: Surgical

INTRODUCTION

Surgical intervention plays a critical role in managing postpartum hemorrhage (PPH) when medical treatments fail to control bleeding. Trauma to the genital tract, such as lacerations or hematomas, requires prompt repair under anesthesia, with surgical exploration or interventional radiology considered for severe cases.

Retained placenta or conditions like placenta accreta may necessitate manual or ultrasound-guided removal. In cases of adherent tissue, surgical techniques, including uterine artery ligation or hysterectomy, may be required to achieve hemostasis and prevent further complications.

Timely transfer to the operating theater enables systematic examination under anesthesia, removal of clots or tissue, and definitive surgical management to ensure maternal safety. This chapter highlights the importance of surgical approaches in addressing life-threatening PPH.

OBSTETRIC TRAUMA

Trauma to the genital tract, such as lacerations or tears, is a common cause of postpartum hemorrhage (PPH), typically leading to venous bleeding. Quick repair of these tears, particularly if arterial bleeding is involved, is crucial. Vulval, preclitoral, or distal vaginal lacerations can also lead to significant blood loss. If a uterine artery laceration is suspected, interventional radiology or surgical exploration with ligation should be considered. Such explorations should be conducted in an operating room under anesthesia. Hematomas, which may present as rectal or pelvic pressure, pain, or deteriorating vital signs, can sometimes develop hours after delivery. If a hematoma is rapidly expanding and vital signs worsen, incision and drainage should be performed, although the source of bleeding may not always be identifiable. Hemostasis can be achieved through suturing or packing.

RETAINED PLACENTA

A history of manual removal of retained placenta (MROP), previous uterine surgery, or other risk factors for morbidly adherent placenta should raise suspicion of retained placenta or placenta accreta. If ultrasound shows a normal endometrial stripe, retained placental tissue is unlikely, but an echogenic mass in the uterus can indicate retained placenta. The first step is to manually remove the placenta under regional anesthesia. If manual removal is unsuccessful, ultrasound-guided removal using large oval forceps may be required, though this carries a risk of perforating the soft, enlarged postpartum uterus. If the placental tissue is adherent to the uterine wall, placenta percreta should be suspected, especially in the presence of risk factors.

SHIFTING TO OPERATION THEATER

If the initial medical management of PPH is unsuccessful, senior medical intervention should be sought for more specialized, secondary measures to stop the bleeding. The patient should be transferred to the operating theater, or if this is not feasible, she should be stabilized and transferred to a referral center, ideally using an anti-shock garment. An examination under anesthesia should be performed to remove any remaining blood clots, placental tissue, or membranes, and the genital tract must be systematically examined for trauma, including the lower vagina, perineum, vaginal side walls, upper vagina, cervix, uterus, and broad ligament.[1]

Tamponade Test

Intrauterine balloon tamponade is commonly employed as a second-line intervention in massive PPH and is a key part of the "HEMOSTASIS" algorithm **(Fig. 1)**. This procedure involves inflating a balloon, such as a Sengstaken–Blakemore **(Fig. 2)**, Rush, Bakri, or condom catheter, in the uterine cavity

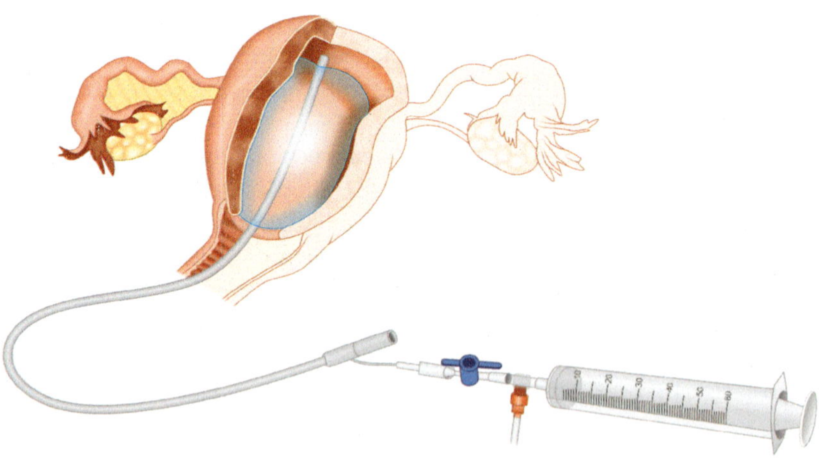

Fig. 1: Intrauterine balloon tamponade.

Sources:

1. Escobar MF, Zambrano MA, Ramos I, Miller S. The Continuous Textbook of Women's Medicine. Global Library of Women's Medicine. 2021.
2. Highmed. Bakri Balloon. [online] Available from https://highmed.am/products/perinatology/bakri-balloon. [Last accessed November, 2024]

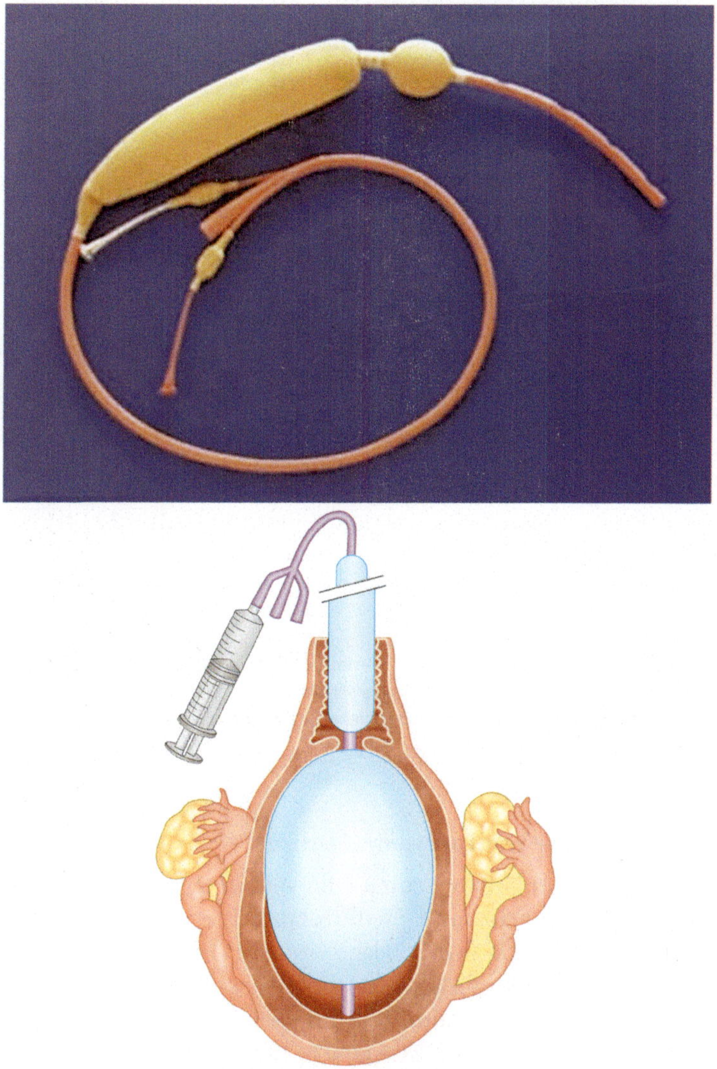

Fig. 2: Sengstaken–Blakemore tube.

to apply mechanical pressure on the placental bed, creating a tamponade effect. The tamponade test helps identify which patients will require further surgical intervention. The test has an 87% sensitivity, meaning that if the bleeding stops after the balloon is inflated, no further surgery will be needed in 87% of cases. The balloon is typically left in place for 4–6 hours before being deflated and removed. In resource-limited settings, if uterine balloons are unavailable, a condom catheter or uterine packing with gauze may be used as alternatives.

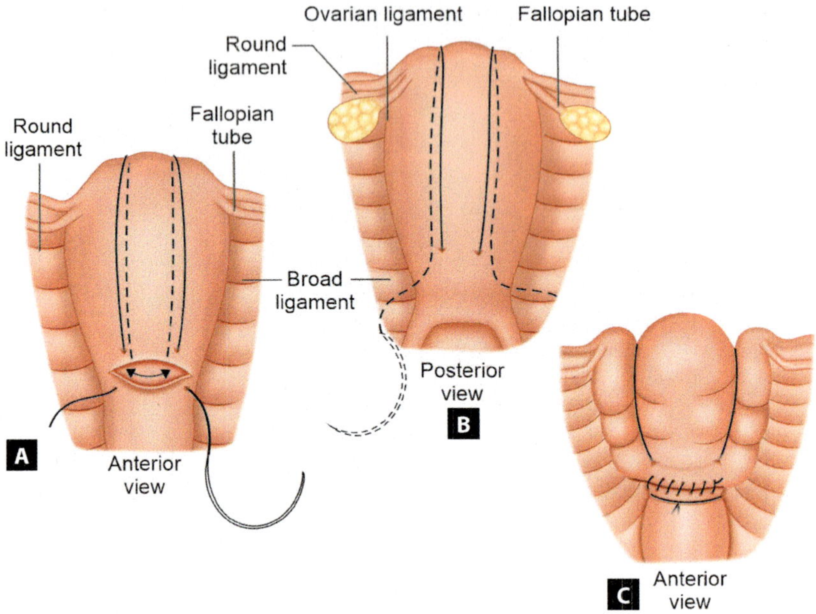

Figs. 3A to C: The B-Lynch brace suture.
Source: Goojha CA, Case A, Pierson R. Development of Asherman syndrome after conservative surgical management of intractable postpartum hemorrhage. [online] Available from https://www.sciencedirect.com/science/article/abs/pii/S0015028210001536. [Last accessed November, 2024]

Hemostatic Uterine Compression Sutures

Uterine compression sutures can be lifesaving in stopping bleeding by compressing the anterior and posterior uterine walls, thereby closing the placental site. The B-Lynch brace suture **(Figs. 3A to C)**, developed for atonic PPH, is commonly used, though several modifications such as vertical and horizontal compression sutures, like Hayman's sutures **(Fig. 4)** have been introduced. The goal of these sutures is to halt bleeding by bringing the uterine walls together. Compression sutures have shown an efficacy rate of 60–75%, with no particular technique proving superior. A study by the UK Obstetric Surveillance System (UKOSS) found a uterine compression suture application rate of 18 per 100,000 deliveries, with a 25% failure rate. The study also highlighted that delays of 2–6 hours between delivery and suture application were associated with a fourfold increase in the likelihood of requiring a hysterectomy, emphasizing the need for timely intervention.

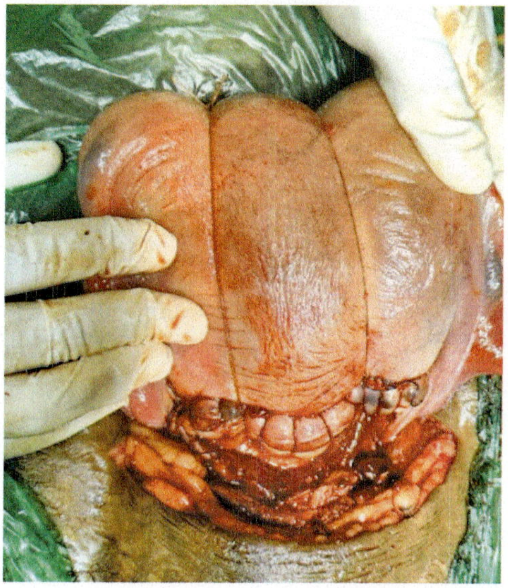

Fig. 4: Hayman suture.
Source: Adapted with permission from Dr NN Chavan, Head of Unit, Department of Obstetrics and Gynaecology, LTMGH, Sion, Mumbai.

SURGICAL METHODS

Systematic Pelvic Devascularization

If bleeding persists despite uterine compression sutures, systematic pelvic devascularization should be considered. This involves ligation of the:

- Uterine artery
- Tubal branch of the ovarian artery
- Internal iliac artery (IIA) in that order

The IIA ligation requires thorough anatomical knowledge to avoid damaging surrounding structures such as the ureters, internal iliac vein, and external iliac vessels. Studies suggest that this procedure rarely impacts future pregnancies and childbirth.

ANATOMY OF INTERNAL ILIAC ARTERY

The aorta is divided into left and right common iliac arteries at the level of the fourth and fifth lumbar vertebra (L4-5) and after a pathway of 4.0–5.0 cm, the common iliac artery gives the branches of external iliac artery and IIA **(Figs. 5 and 6)**. The IIA runs inferno-medially after the pelvic brim and has two divisions—posterior and anterior. The anterior division starts after

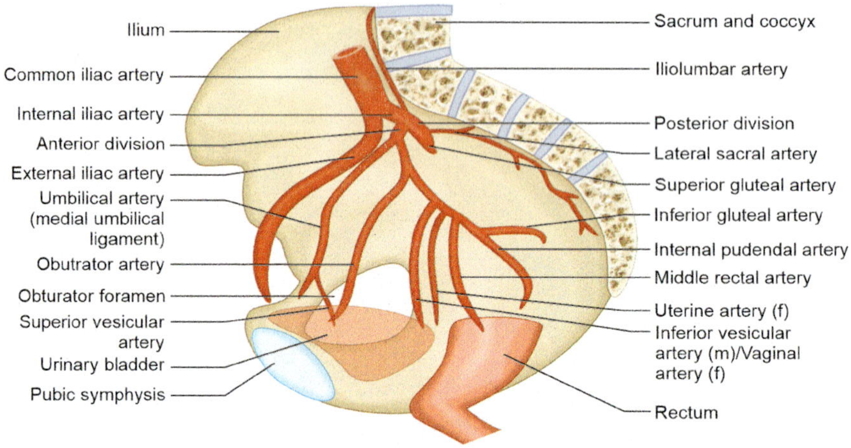

Fig. 5: Anatomy of internal iliac artery.
Source: Ditki. Arteries - Internal Iliac & Branches. [online] Available from https://ditki.com/course/gross-anatomy/glossary/gross-anatomic-microscopic-structure/arteries-internal-iliac-branches. [Last accessed November, 2024]

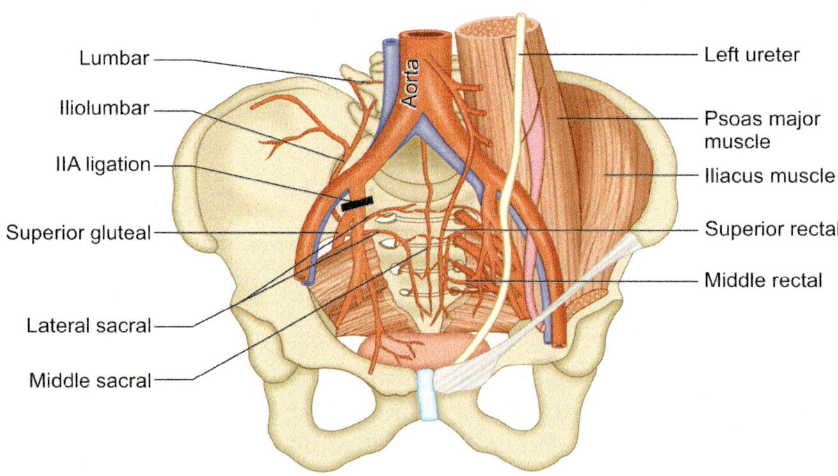

Fig. 6: Anatomy and relations of internal iliac artery. (IIA: internal iliac artery)
Source: Bleich AT, Rahn DD, Wieslander CK, Wai CY, Roshanravan SM, Corton MM. Posterior division of the internal iliac artery: Anatomic variations and clinical applications. Am J Obstet Gynecol. 2007;197(6):658.e1-5.

3.5–5.0 cm from the origin of the IIA and branches of the posterior division diverge before that part. The anterior division is the main blood supply of the pelvic viscera **(Table 1)**.

RELATIONS TO INTERNAL ILIAC ARTERY

Table 2 highlights the anatomic relations of IIA.

INDICATION OF INTERNAL ILIAC ARTERY LIGATION

Box 1 describes the various indications for ligation of IIA.

TABLE 1: Branches of internal iliac artery.

Anterior division	*Posterior division*
Internal pudendal artery	Iliolumbar artery
Inferior gluteal artery	Lateral sacral artery
Obturator artery	Superior gluteal artery
Uterine artery	
Middle rectal artery	
Vaginal artery	
Superior vesical artery	
Inferior vesical artery	

Source: Selçuk İ, Uzuner B, Boduç E, Baykuş Y, Akar B, Güngör T. Step-by-step ligation of the internal iliac artery. J Turk Ger Gynecol Assoc. 2019;20(2):123-8.

TABLE 2: Relations to internal iliac artery.

Anterior	Peritoneum
Medial	Ureter
Inferomedial	Internal iliac vein
Lateral	Psoas major and internal obturator muscle
Inferolateral	Obturator nerve

Source: Selçuk İ, Uzuner B, Boduç E, Baykuş Y, Akar B, Güngör T. Step-by-step ligation of the internal iliac artery. J Turk Ger Gynecol Assoc. 2019;20(2):123-8.

BOX 1: Indication of internal iliac artery ligation.

Obstetric factors:
- Uterine atony
- Uterine laceration or rupture
- Abruptio placenta
- Placental adhesion disorders
- Placenta accreta, increta, percreta
- Cervical pregnancy

Gynaecological factors:
- Gynaecologic oncologic procedures
- Mass/tumor at deeper part of pelvis
- Exenteration surgery
- Radical hysterectomy
- Extended radical operations

Postoperative unknown site for pelvic hemorrhage

Source: Selçuk İ, Uzuner B, Boduç E, Baykuş Y, Akar B, Güngör T. Step-by-step ligation of the internal iliac artery. J Turk Ger Gynecol Assoc. 2019;20(2):123-8.

PROBABLE OPERATIVE COMPLICATIONS DUE TO INTERNAL ILIAC ARTERY LIGATION

- Injury to external iliac vein
- Injury to internal iliac vein
- Ligation or laceration of the external iliac artery
- Ligation or laceration of the ureter

Interventional Radiology

Pelvic arterial embolization is an option for stable patients with ongoing slow bleeding after primary interventions have failed. It may also be indicated when surgical interventions are ineffective (e.g., for uterine arteriovenous malformations or broad ligament hematomas). WHO guidelines recommend uterine artery embolization (UAE) as a second-line treatment for PPH caused by uterine atony, though the quality of supporting evidence is low **(Fig. 7)**. Success rates for pelvic arterial embolization range from 86 to 100%.

Despite the effectiveness, UAE is associated with potential complications, including endometritis, intrauterine adhesions (synechiae), and rare but serious risks such as embolus migration, uterine or bladder wall necrosis, and vaginal fistula.

There are also risks of IIA perforation and inadvertent occlusion of the external iliac artery, which can lead to lower limb ischemia. Studies indicate that future fertility is not significantly compromised by UAE, despite a reported incidence of uterine synechiae in 11.7% of cases. Additionally,

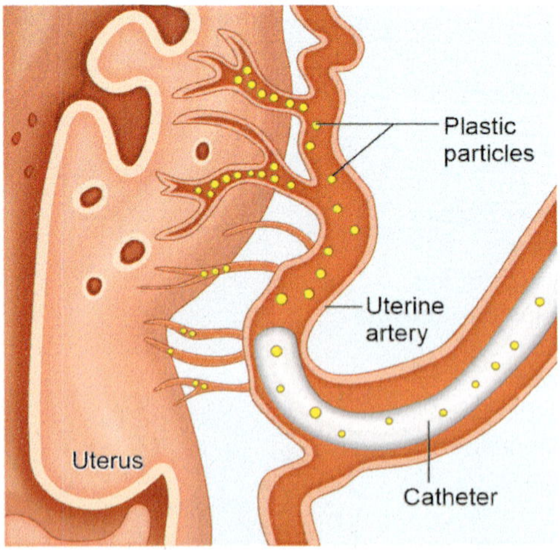

Fig. 7: Principle of uterine artery embolization.
Source: Sydney Fibroid Clinic. FAQs about Uterine Artery Embolization (UAE). [online] Available from https://www.sydneyfibroidclinic.com.au/adenomyosis/adenomyosis-faqs/. [Last accessed November, 2024]

rates of preterm birth (5–15%) and fetal growth restriction (7%) after UAE are comparable to the general obstetric population.

Peripartum Hysterectomy

Peripartum hysterectomy is a lifesaving measure in cases of massive PPH, but it should be performed at the appropriate time. If conservative methods could still be effective, premature hysterectomy may increase maternal morbidity and mortality and result in future infertility. For this reason, a second consultant should be involved in the decision to proceed with peripartum hysterectomy. A recent systematic review found that the most common causes of hysterectomy were abnormal placentation (38%), uterine atony (29%), and uterine rupture (12%). Subtotal hysterectomy is technically quicker and easier to perform, but a total hysterectomy is preferable when the cause of PPH is located in the lower uterine segment, such as with placenta previa, lower uterine segment rupture, or cervical trauma, or in cases of morbidly adherent placenta.[2]

REFERENCES

1. Escobar MF, Nassar AH, Theron G, Barnea ER, Nicholson W, Ramasauskaite D, et al. FIGO recommendations on the management of postpartum hemorrhage 2022. Int J Gynaecol Obstet. 2022;157 Suppl 1(Suppl 1):3-50.
2. Mousa HA, Blum J, Abou El Senoun G, Shakur H, Alfirevic Z. Treatment for primary postpartum haemorrhage. Cochrane Database Syst Rev. 2014;2014(2):CD003249.

6

CHAPTER

Chavan's Internal Iliac Artery Ligation Forceps

INTRODUCTION AND DESCRIPTION OF THE CHAVAN'S INTERNAL ILIAC ARTERY LIGATION FORCEPS

The procedure of internal iliac artery ligation using a forceps with two eyes at the end is a surgical technique employed to control pelvic hemorrhage, often in cases like postpartum hemorrhage or pelvic trauma. After proper exposure of the retroperitoneal space, the surgeon identifies the internal iliac artery. A specially designed forceps, with its curved design and specialized end having two eyes, is used to carefully isolate the artery **(Figs. 1A and B)**. The eyes at the end of the forceps allow for easy threading of the ligature, typically a nonabsorbable suture. The suture is passed through the eyes, wrapped around the artery, and securely tied, ensuring minimal risk of slippage. This reduces blood flow to the pelvis while preserving the external iliac artery for continued blood supply to the lower extremities. The procedure requires precision to avoid damaging adjacent structures like veins or nerves and is an essential step in controlling life-threatening hemorrhages.

STEPS OF INTERNAL ILIAC ARTERY LIGATION

Step 1: Access the Retroperitoneum

There are many ways to access the retroperitoneum in the pelvis. It can be accessed by dividing the round ligament followed by opening the leaves of broad ligament, revealing the retroperitoneal space. More access to the retroperitoneal structures can be sought by opening the broad ligament in a cephalad direction, lateral and parallel to the infundibulopelvic ligament.

Step 2: Dissect the Pararectal Space

Dissection of this avascular potential space is carried out in a craniocaudal direction, parallel to the course of the great vessels. The dissection in this space must occur medial to the psoas muscle.

The use of a narrow Deaver with cephalad traction is critical to optimize visualization and identify the borders of this space. The pararectal space is bordered by the sacrum posteriorly, the internal iliac artery laterally, the cardinal ligament anteriorly, and the ureter medially.

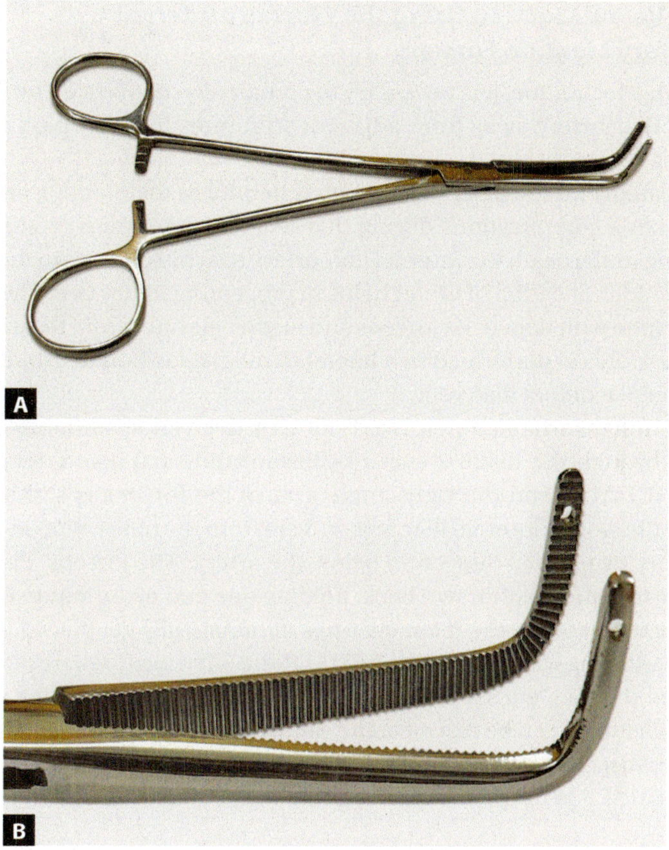

Figs. 1A and B: Chavan's internal iliac artery ligation forceps.

Step 3: Identify the Anatomy

After dissecting the pararectal space, it is necessary to identify key anatomic structures.

The external iliac vein courses are deep to the external iliac artery, just adjacent to the internal iliac artery. The ureter runs along the medial leaf of the broad ligament within the pararectal space. It can be seen vermiculating here. The ureter runs along the medial leaf of broad ligament.

Step 4: Isolate the Internal Iliac Artery

After identifying relevant landmarks, the internal iliac artery is isolated by dissecting away the surrounding connective tissue. Note the proximity of the adjacent external iliac artery and vein. Care must be taken to avoid injury to these structures during the dissection.

Step 5: Vessel Ligation Using the Chavan's Internal Iliac Artery Ligation Forceps

During this technique, it is necessary to completely mobilize a portion of the internal iliac artery away from adjacent structures to safely pass a ligature around it.

Repeatedly identifying the anatomy is helpful in maintaining orientation and avoiding complications during this step. Utmost care is required when dissecting underneath the internal iliac artery to avoid damage to the internal iliac vein. Identification of ureter helps in preventing injury to it. The vessel is then grasped with Babcock's forceps and further elevated from the underlying structures. This is performed in a lateral to medial fashion to avoid injury to the adjacent external iliac vein.

Two nonabsorbable linen No. 1 sutures/delayed absorbable No. 1 are loaded through the distal 2 eyes of Chavan's internal iliac artery ligation forceps (CIIALF) and the right-angle arm of the forceps is slid below the anterior division of internal iliac artery, 3 cm from the bifurcation of common iliac artery by gradual dissection below the artery. The forceps' distal right-angled arm is then withdrawn back, holding one end of the suture by 2 small artery forceps, so that the linen ligatures automatically get placed below the vessel. Following withdrawal of the CIIALF, the linen ligatures are placed 1 cm apart and the long ends are cut short. The advantage of using the CIIALF is that two ligatures can be placed at the same time on the vessel, thus reducing repetitive insertion and withdrawal of instrument.

The CIIALF is in the process of getting patented by the Government of India.

7

CHAPTER

Recent Advances in Management of Postpartum Hemorrhage

RECENT ADVANCES

- *Conservative surgical techniques:* New techniques for managing placenta percreta, such as the Triple-P procedure, offer alternatives to peripartum hysterectomy and have shown promise in reducing blood loss and avoiding hysterectomy.
- *Topical hemostatic agents:* The use of topical agents to enhance hemostasis is becoming more prevalent, aiding in the management of bleeding.
- *Tranexamic acid (TXA):* TXA has been shown to significantly reduce deaths due to bleeding when administered within 3 hours of delivery. Its inclusion in recent guidelines reflects its importance in postpartum hemorrhage (PPH) management.
- *Transfusion strategies:* Changes in blood product transfusion ratios, such as the 1:1:1 ratio of fresh frozen plasma (FFP): platelets.

These advancements in the management of PPH are crucial in addressing this persistent challenge and improving outcomes for affected women.

TRANSFUSION STRATEGIES

Fluid replacement: Initially, crystalloids and colloids are used to manage blood volume, but they can worsen coagulopathy and enhance fibrinolysis. Current practice emphasizes correcting coagulopathy by increasing the ratio of FFP to red blood cells (RBCs) to improve survival rates. A 1:1:1 ratio of FFP:platelets:RBCs has been shown to significantly reduce mortality compared to traditional ratios.

MASSIVE TRANSFUSION/TRAUMA EXSANGUINATION PROTOCOLS

Protocol-driven early transfusion: New protocols advocate for the early, coordinated use of RBCs, platelets, FFP, and crystalloids. This approach addresses the triad of hypothermia, acidosis, and coagulopathy and aims to improve outcomes. However, optimal pathways for obstetric patients are still under discussion, and protocols are often adapted from trauma care guidelines.

CELL SALVAGE

Emerging use: Cell salvage has traditionally been limited in obstetrics due to concerns about alloimmunization and amniotic fluid embolism. However, with improved filter systems and its potential role in managing morbidly invasive placentas, its use is being re-evaluated. It is recommended for caesarean sections or laparotomies rather than vaginal deliveries.

USE OF FIBRINOGEN

Fibrinogen levels: Transfusion practices are shifting toward maintaining fibrinogen levels, with recommendations suggesting a minimum of 200 mg/dL to manage ongoing bleeding. Cryoprecipitate and fibrinogen concentrates are used, with varying practices depending on regional guidelines.

ANTIFIBRINOLYTICS (FIG. 1)

Tranexamic acid (TXA): TXA has been found effective in reducing bleeding-related deaths in PPH, particularly if administered within 3 hours of delivery. Despite its efficacy, its use should be time-sensitive, and further studies are needed to refine its application in obstetric hemorrhage.

LABORATORY TESTING

Fibrinogen and viscoelastic testing: Fibrinogen levels are crucial for assessing PPH severity, with levels below 200 mg/dL indicating severe bleeding. Viscoelastic tests like thromboelastography (TEG) and rotational thromboelastometry (ROTEM) are gaining popularity for their rapid assessment of clot formation and dissolution, offering more immediate guidance for transfusion needs.

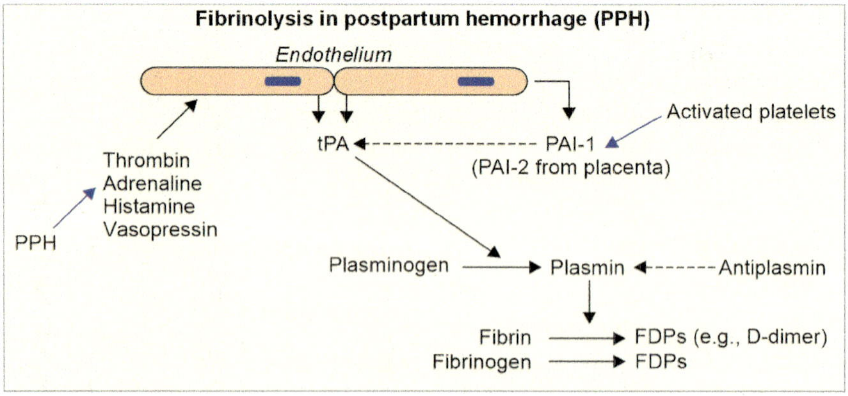

Fig. 1: Mechanism of antifibrinolytics. (FDP: fibrin degradation product; PAI: plasminogen activator inhibitor; tPA: tissue plasminogen activator)

Source: Hibbs SP, Roberts I, Shakur-Still H, Hunt BJ. Post-partum haemorrhage and tranexamic acid: A global issue. Br J Haematol. 2018;180(6):799-807.

RECOMBINANT FACTOR VIIA AND PROTHROMBIN COMPLEX CONCENTRATE

- *Concentrate recombinant factor VIIa:* Used in hemophilia and experimental settings for severe obstetric hemorrhage, though its role remains uncertain and requires careful consideration due to potential thromboembolic risks.
- *Prothrombin complex concentrates (PCCs):* These are used for reversing anticoagulation but are not yet well-established in obstetric hemorrhage management.

TRIPLE-P PROCEDURE

Conservative surgical approach: The Triple-P procedure offers an alternative to peripartum hysterectomy for placental percreta. It involves:

- Placental localization
- Pelvic devascularization
- Myometrial excision with uterine wall reconstruction

Initial reports suggest reduced blood loss and avoidance of hysterectomy in some cases.

These advancements aim to improve the management of PPH, reduce morbidity and mortality, and adapt transfusion practices to better address the challenges of massive bleeding.[1]

POSTPARTUM HEMORRHAGE BUNDLE (FIG. 2)

Bundles are a newer concept in providing optimal, comprehensive healthcare. They are formulated. All evidences are put together, in order to develop a strategy for dealing with a crucial cause of concern, and that works in all health care settings, in all income countries and in urban, semi-urban, and rural areas.[2]

Several bundles tried but the two universally accepted and being intensively researched:

1. E-MOTIVE
2. PPH EMC bundle

The E-MOTIVE trial: This is a multi-country, parallel cluster randomized trial with a baseline control phase, along with mixed-methods and health economic evaluations. It aims at evaluating the implementation of early detection and the usage of WHO MOTIVE. It aims to explore the clinical, implementational, and resource outcomes.[3]

The E-MOTIVE bundle mainly consists of three components **(Fig. 3)**:

1. A strategy for early detection of PPH, triggering the "first response" treatment bundle

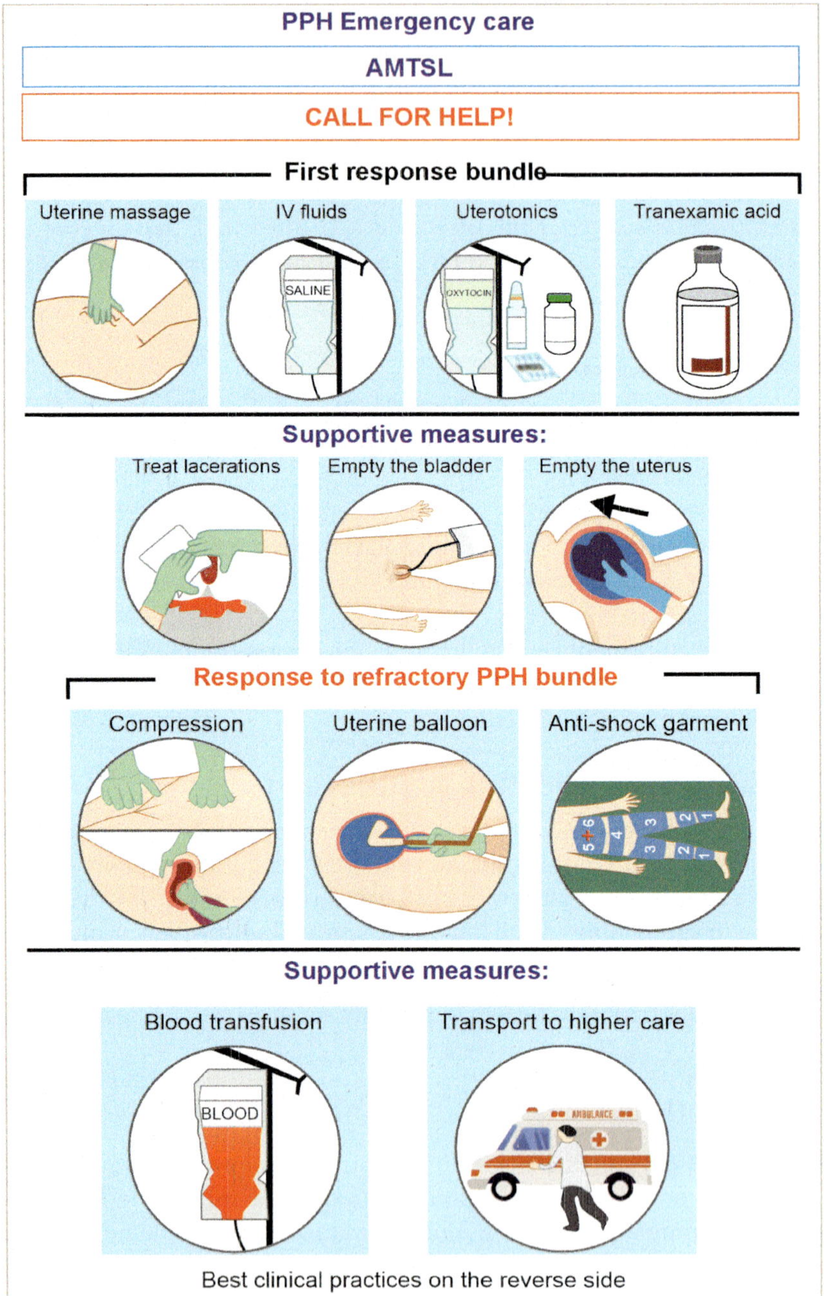

Fig. 2: The PPH care bundle. (PPH: postpartum hemorrhage)
Source: FIGO. PPH Emergency Care Using a Bundle Approach (PPH EmC). [online] Available from https://www.jhpiego.org/wp-content/uploads/2020/07/MGH-PPH-EmC-Executive-Summary_July-2020.pdf. [Last accessed November, 2024]

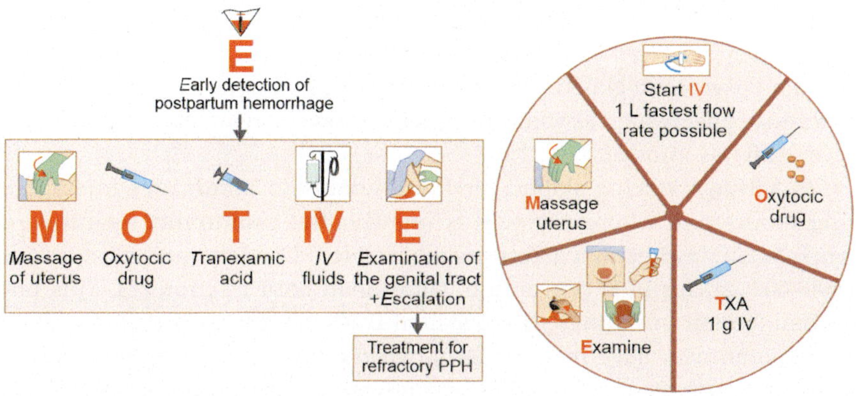

Fig. 3: The components of E-MOTIVE bundle.
Source: Forbes G, Akter S, Miller S, Galadanci H, Qureshi Z, Fawcus S, et al. Factors influencing postpartum haemorrhage detection and management and the implementation of a new postpartum haemorrhage care bundle (E-MOTIVE) in Kenya, Nigeria, and South Africa. Implement Sci. 2023;18(1):1.

2. "First response" bundle called "MOTIVE", based on the WHO guideline recommendations and consisting of:
   - Uterine massage
   - Oxytocic drugs
   - Tranexamic acid
   - IV fluids
   - Examination and escalation
3. An implementation strategy, focusing on simulation-based training, peer-assisted learning, local E-MOTIVE champions, feedback of actionable data to providers, calibrated drape with action line, and MOTIVE emergency kits

FIGO RECOMMENDATIONS 2022 FOR PREVENTION AND TREATMENT OF PPH

Prevention Guidelines

Recommendations for preventing PPH during the third stage of labor include the use of uterotonics for all deliveries. Oxytocin, administered intravenously or intramuscularly at a dosage of 10 IU, is advised for preventing PPH in both vaginal and caesarean deliveries. In places where oxytocin is utilized, it is crucial to maintain the integrity of the cold chain for oxytocin storage. In situations where oxytocin is either unavailable or its quality cannot be assured, alternative injectable uterotonics such as ergometrine/methylergometrine (200 µg IM/IV, provided hypertensive disorders are safely ruled out), oral misoprostol (400–600 µg), or carbetocin (100 µg IM/IV) are recommended for PPH prevention.[4,5]

Combining ergometrine with oxytocin or misoprostol with oxytocin might offer enhanced efficacy in preventing PPH ≥500 mL compared to the standard oxytocin regimen. However, these combinations carry a higher risk of adverse effects such as vomiting and hypertension with ergometrine, and fever with misoprostol.

In settings lacking skilled birth attendants to administer injectable uterotonics and where oxytocin is unavailable, community health care workers and lay health workers are advised to administer oral misoprostol (400–600 μg) for PPH prevention. Controlled cord traction (CCT) is not recommended in settings where skilled birth attendants are unavailable. For women who have received prophylactic oxytocin, sustained uterine massage is not recommended as an intervention for preventing PPH. It is recommended to assess postpartum abdominal uterine tonus early for identifying uterine atony in all women.

For preventing PPH in caesarean deliveries, the recommended method for placental removal is oxytocin administration (IV or IM) combined with CCT.

Treatment Guidelines

Intravenous oxytocin is the preferred initial uterotonic medication for managing PPH. If intravenous oxytocin is unavailable or ineffective, alternative options such as intramuscular ergometrine, oxytocin-ergometrine fixed dose, or prostaglandin drugs (including sublingual misoprostol—800 μg) are recommended. There is insufficient evidence regarding the safety and effectiveness of administering an additional 800-μg dose of misoprostol for treating PPH in women who have already received 600 μg of prophylactic misoprostol orally.[4]

For the initial intravenous fluid resuscitation of women with PPH, isotonic crystalloids are preferred over colloids. Early administration of intravenous TXA, within 3 hours of birth and upon diagnosis of PPH, in addition to standard care, is recommended for women experiencing clinically diagnosed PPH following vaginal or caesarean delivery. TXA should be administered at a rate of 1 g (100 mg/mL) intravenously over 10 minutes, with a second dose of 1 g intravenously if bleeding persists after 30 minutes or if bleeding resumes within 24 hours of the first dose. Expanding the use of TXA for PPH treatment could positively impact health equity and outcomes, particularly for disadvantaged women, especially in low- and middle-income countries.

Uterine massage is recommended as part of PPH treatment. In cases of uterine atony after vaginal birth, bimanual uterine compression or external aortic compression is advised as a temporary measure until appropriate care is available. If uterotonics fail or are unavailable, uterine balloon tamponade is recommended as an effective nonsurgical technique, following the exclusion of retained products of conception or uterine rupture.[5] The nonpneumatic antishock garment is also recommended as a temporary measure until appropriate care can be provided. However, uterine packing is not recommended for treating PPH due to uterine atony after vaginal birth.[6]

Uterine artery embolization can be considered as a conservative management option for PPH if technical resources and skilled personnel are available. If bleeding persists despite conservative interventions, surgical interventions such as compression suture techniques, uterine and hypogastric artery ligation, and hysterectomy are recommended.[7] The primary aim is to halt bleeding before coagulation abnormalities and organ damage occur, with conservative measures attempted initially and more invasive procedures pursued if necessary.

Flowchart 1 shows treatment algorithm for management of PPH.

WHO road map: The creation of the WHO road map stemmed from a thorough scientific examination of PPH status across four critical domains: research, norms and standards, implementation, and advocacy. Valuable insights were gathered through online and face-to-face discussions involving a diverse group of stakeholders operating at both international and country levels. To ensure the strength and inclusivity of each domain, a meticulous multi-step process was employed to autonomously delineate forthcoming agendas for all four strategic areas, thereby capturing the collective consensus of the global community on essential priorities for collaborative action.

NEW DRUGS ON THE BLOCK

Carbetocin

Carbetocin, a synthetic oxytocin analog, was initially characterized in 1987. It features a half-life of 40 minutes, approximately 4–10 times longer than oxytocin. Upon intravenous administration of an optimal dosage of 100 μg, uterine contractions typically commence in <2 minutes. It is suggested that a single dose of carbetocin may simulate the effects of a 16-hour intravenous oxytocin infusion, contributing to heightened uterine tone and diminished risk of PPH in elective caesarean sections.[8]

WOMAN Trial 2017: Tranexamic Acid

In this randomized, double-blind, placebo-controlled trial, women aged 16 years and older diagnosed with PPH following either vaginal birth or caesarean section were recruited from 193 hospitals across 21 countries. Participants were randomly allocated to receive either 1 g of intravenous TXA or a matching placebo alongside standard care. If bleeding persisted after 30 minutes or stopped and then resumed within 24 hours of the initial dose, a second dose of 1 g of TXA or placebo could be administered.[1] TXA decreases death due to blood loss owing to PPH. No adverse effects have been noted. It is recommended to give TXA as soon as possible when bleeding ensues or at least within 3 hours.

Flowchart 1: Management algorithm of PPH.

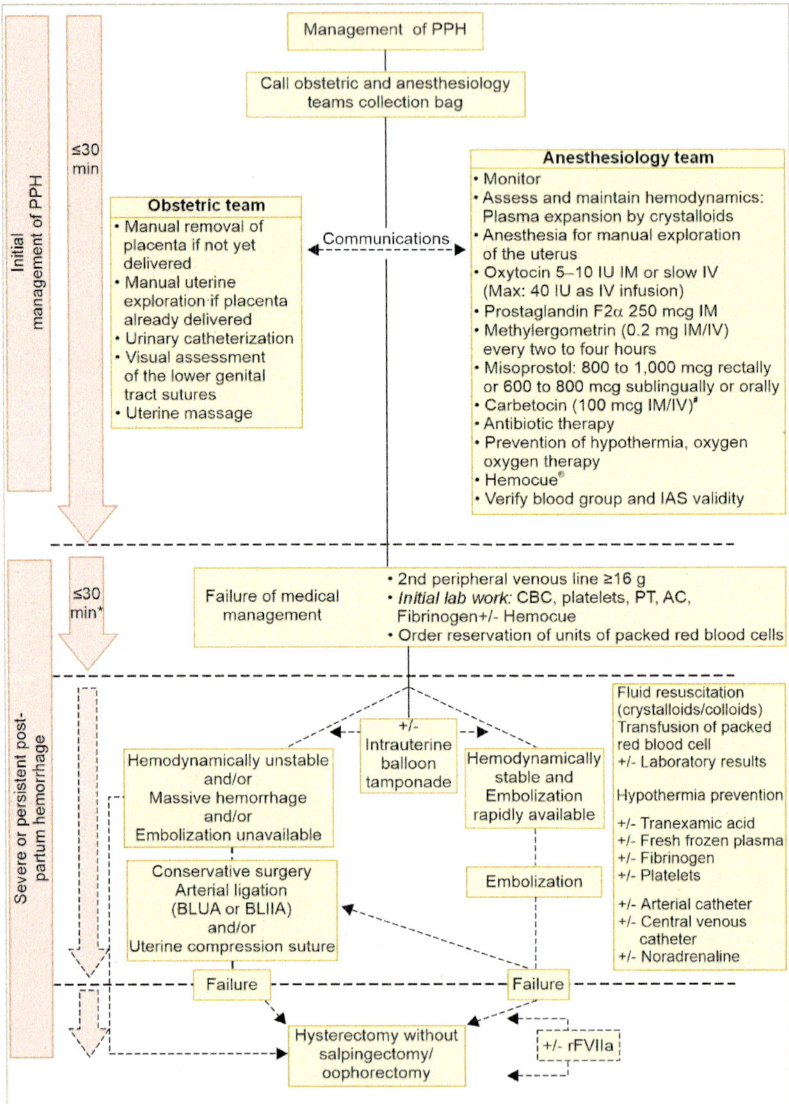

*For general guidance, to be adapted according to the quantity of bleeding.

#Under trial PPH.

(PPH: postpartum hemorrhage; Min: minute; slow IV: slow intravenous; IM: intramuscular; IU: international unit; IAS: irregular antibody screening; BLUA: bilateral ligation of the uterine arteries; BLIIA: bilateral ligation of the internal iliac arteries; CBC: complete blood count; PT: prothrombin time; ACT: activated clotting time; rFVIIa: recombinant activated Factor VII)

Source: Sentilhes L, Vayssière C, Deneux-Tharaux C, Aya AG, Bayoumeu F, Bonnet MP, et al. Postpartum haemorrhage: guidelines for clinical practice from the French College of Gynaecologists and Obstetricians (CNGOF): in collaboration with the French Society of Anesthesiology and Intensive Care (SFAR). Eur J Obstet Gynecol Reprod Biol. 2016;198:12-21.

Fibrinogen Concentrate

Fibrinogen is one of the best predictors for blood loss. Levels <1 g/L should trigger transfusions. Fibrinogen concentrates are used to decrease the need of transfusion of packed red blood cells, FFP, and platelet concentrates. This, further, decreased the risk associated with transfusion and its reactions.[6]

Recombinant Factor VII

One of the recent and innovative advancements in PPH management involves the utilization of recombinant activated factor VII (rFVIIa). Initially developed for treating bleeding episodes in patients with hemophilia A or B, rFVIIa has found broader application beyond its recognized indications. It has been effectively employed "off-label" on an empirical basis in managing massive PPH. Since its first reported usage almost a decade ago in obstetric hemorrhage, rFVIIa has demonstrated remarkable efficacy and has played a vital role in saving numerous lives. Over the past decade, several case reports and series have documented successful PPH management using rFVIIa.[9]

REFERENCES

1. WOMAN Trial Collaborators. Effect of early tranexamic acid administration on mortality, hysterectomy, and other morbidities in women with post-partum haemorrhage (WOMAN): an international, randomised, double-blind, placebo-controlled trial. Lancet Lond Engl. 2017;389(10084):2105-16.
2. Lavallée JF, Gray TA, Dumville J, Russell W, Cullum N. The effects of care bundles on patient outcomes: a systematic review and meta-analysis. Implement Sci IS. 2017;12(1):142.
3. Gallos I, Devall A, Martin J, Middleton L, Beeson L, Galadanci H, et al. Randomized Trial of Early Detection and Treatment of Postpartum Hemorrhage. N Engl J Med. 2023;389(1):11-21.
4. Escobar MF, Nassar AH, Theron G, Barnea ER, Nicholson W, Ramasauskaite D, et al. FIGO recommendations on the management of postpartum hemorrhage 2022. Int J Gynaecol Obstet. 2022;157 Suppl 1(Suppl 1):3-50.
5. Tindell K, Garfinkel R, Abu-Haydar E, Ahn R, Burke TF, Conn K, et al. Uterine balloon tamponade for the treatment of postpartum haemorrhage in resource-poor settings: a systematic review. BJOG Int J Obstet Gynaecol. 2013;120(1):5-14.
6. Kumaraswami S, Butwick A. Latest advances in postpartum hemorrhage management. Best Pract Res Clin Anaesthesiol. 2022;36(1):123-34.
7. Mousa HA, Blum J, Abou El Senoun G, Shakur H, Alfirevic Z. Treatment for primary postpartum haemorrhage. Cochrane Database Syst Rev. 2014;2014(2):CD003249.
8. Larciprete G, Montagnoli C, Frigo M, Panetta V, Todde C, Zuppani B, et al. Carbetocin versus oxytocin in caesarean section with high risk of post-partum haemorrhage. J Prenat Med. 2013;7(1):12-8.
9. Magon N, Babu KM, Kapur K, Chopra S, Joneja GS. Recombinant activated factor VII in postpartum haemorrhage. Niger Med J. 2013;54(5):289-94.

CHAPTER 8

Multiple Choice Questions

1. **Which of the following is the definition of primary postpartum hemorrhage (PPH) as per ACOG guidelines?**
   a. Blood loss >250 mL within 24 hours after delivery
   b. Blood loss >500 mL after vaginal delivery or >1,000 mL after caesarean section within 24 hours
   c. Hemoglobin drop of 2 g/dL within 48 hours after delivery
   d. Blood loss requiring transfusion within 7 days of delivery

Ans. b. Blood loss >500 mL after vaginal delivery or >1,000 mL after caesarean section within 24 hours

2. **Which of the following is not included in the "4 T's" of PPH etiology?**
   a. Tone (uterine atony)
   b. Tissue (retained products of conception)
   c. Trauma (genital tract injury)
   d. Thrombocytopenia

Ans. d. Thrombocytopenia

3. **Uterotonics are first-line agents in managing PPH. Which of the following is contraindicated in a patient with pre-eclampsia or hypertension?**
   a. Oxytocin
   b. Misoprostol
   c. Ergometrine
   d. Carboprost

Ans. c. Ergometrine

4. **Tranexamic acid, as per WHO guidelines, should be administered for PPH within what time frame to be most effective?**
   a. Within 15 minutes of diagnosis
   b. Within 3 hours of delivery
   c. Within 6 hours of delivery
   d. Anytime during the postpartum period

Ans. b. Within 3 hours of delivery

5. Which of the following surgical techniques is considered the most fertility-preserving in managing refractory PPH?

a. Uterine artery embolization
b. B-Lynch compression suture
c. Peripartum hysterectomy
d. Internal iliac artery ligation

Ans. b. B-Lynch compression suture

6. Which diagnostic parameter is considered the earliest reliable indicator of significant blood loss in PPH?

a. Hemoglobin levels
b. Tachycardia
c. Drop in systolic blood pressure
d. Pallor

Ans. b. Tachycardia

7. What is the first-line approach for uterine atony unresponsive to medical management in a hemodynamically stable patient?

a. Hysterectomy
b. Internal iliac artery ligation
c. Uterine balloon tamponade
d. B-Lynch suture

Ans. c. Uterine balloon tamponade

8. Which of the following uterotonic drugs is contraindicated in a patient with a history of asthma?

a. Oxytocin
b. Ergometrine
c. Carboprost (15-methyl PGF2α)
d. Misoprostol

Ans. c. Carboprost (15-methyl PGF2α)

9. Internal iliac artery ligation is primarily performed in PPH to:

a. Decrease systemic blood pressure
b. Reduce pelvic blood flow by 85%
c. Increase uterine perfusion
d. Prevent coagulopathy

Ans. b. Reduce pelvic blood flow by 85%

10. The success rate of internal iliac artery ligation in controlling pelvic hemorrhage is approximately:

a. 50–60%
b. 70–80%
c. 80–90%
d. >90%

Ans. c. 80–90%

11. Which of the following is a key landmark for identifying the internal iliac artery during ligation?

a. Uterine artery
b. Common iliac artery bifurcation
c. Inferior epigastric artery
d. Round ligament of the uterus

Ans. b. Common iliac artery bifurcation

12. Which vessel is directly spared during internal iliac artery ligation?

a. External iliac artery
b. Uterine artery
c. Superior gluteal artery
d. Superior vesical artery

Ans. c. Superior gluteal artery

13. What is the primary indication for internal iliac artery ligation in obstetrics?

a. Broad ligament hematoma
b. Refractory PPH unresponsive to medical and conservative surgical management
c. Severe pre-eclampsia with HELLP syndrome
d. Uterine inversion

Ans. b. Refractory PPH unresponsive to medical and conservative surgical management

14. During internal iliac artery ligation, care must be taken to avoid injury to which structure lying anterior to the artery?

a. Ureter
b. Ovarian vein
c. Inferior mesenteric vein
d. Psoas muscle

Ans. a. Ureter

15. Which of the following complications is least likely after internal iliac artery ligation?

a. Ischemic necrosis of pelvic organs
b. Ureteral injury
c. Temporary reduction in fertility
d. Neuropathy of the obturator nerve

Ans. c. Temporary reduction in fertility

Index

Page numbers followed by *b* refer to box, *f* refer to figure, *fc* refer to flowchart, and *t* refer to table.

U

V

W